ARTHUR RACKHAM'S BOOK OF PICTURES

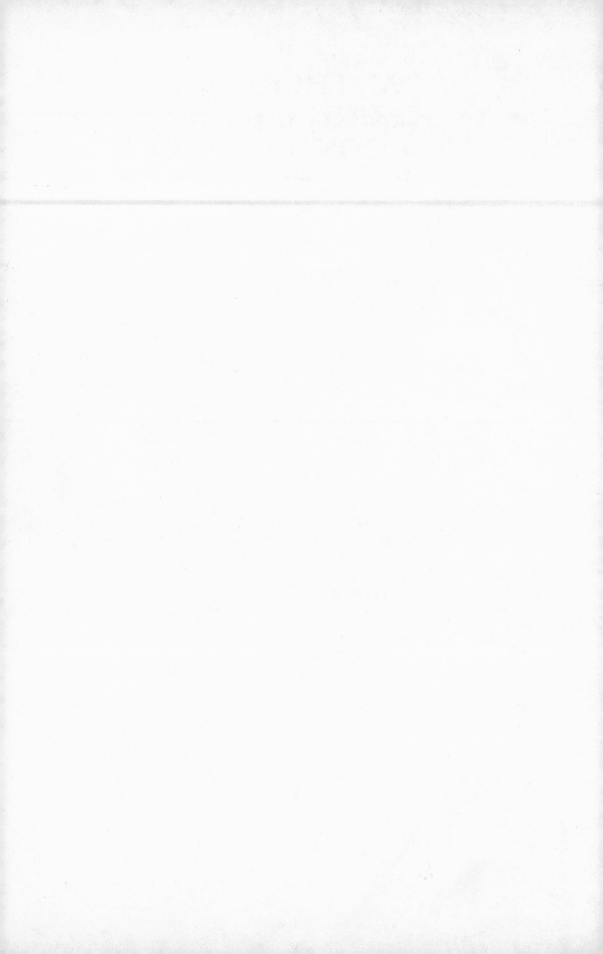

ARTHUR RACKHAM'S BOOK OF PICTURES

WITH AN INTRODUCTION BY SIR ARTHUR QUILLER-COUCH

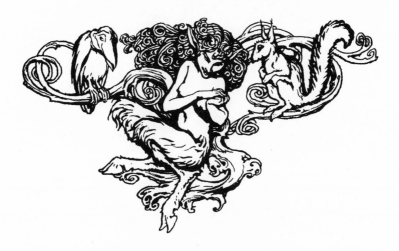

WITH A NEW FOREWORD BY
ELIZABETH CONGDON KOVANEN

AVENEL BOOKS
NEW YORK

NOTE

A FEW of the illustrations in this book have
been published before in magazines or periodi-
cals ; in most cases as first sketches in black
and white only.   These have since been carried
out as pictures, and in that form are reproduced
here for the first time.   In this connection my
thanks are due to the proprietors of the *Ladies'*
Field and the *Pall Mall Magazine.*   I am also
much indebted to the owners of several of the
pictures who have so kindly allowed me to
borrow them for reproduction.

A. R.

Special material copyright © MCMLXXIX by Crown Publishers, Inc.
All rights reserved.
This edition is published by Avenel Books,
distributed by Crown Publishers, Inc.
a b c d e f g h
AVENEL 1979 EDITION
Manufactured in the United States of America

Library of Congress Cataloging in Publication Data

Rackham, Arthur, 1867-1939.
  Arthur Rackham's Book of pictures.

  Reprint of the 1913 ed. published by W. Heinemann,
London.
  1. Rackham, Arthur, 1867-1939. I. Title.
II. Title: Book of pictures.
NC242.R3A4 1979   741.9'42   79-17257
ISBN 0-517-29763-9

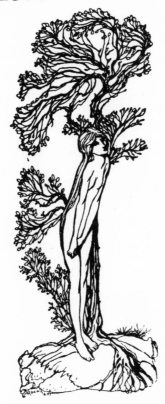

FOREWORD

Arthur Rackham is said to have kept the fairy world alive for children of the twentieth century. And children need fairies, says Arthur Quiller-Couch, to account for the marvels that are happening around them all the time. "How else can we explain toadstools?" he asks!

Born in London in 1867, the fourth of twelve children, Rackham, at age seventeen, enrolled as an evening student in the Lambeth School of Art. After working during the day for eight years as a clerk in the Westminster Fire Office, he became a full-time artist on the staff of the *Westminster Budget*. In 1903, he married Edyth Starkie, also an artist; in 1908, his daughter Barbara was born, and, in that same year, he became a member of the Royal Water-Color Society.

Essentially a graphic journalist in his early years, the young artist showed little of the imaginative genius that was to emerge later, although he developed an eye for detail and an integrity of line that was to be characteristic of his future work. The first flowering of his fanciful style was *The Dolly Dialogues*, published in 1894. It is speculated that his seemingly overnight transformation from a good journalist-artist to the prolific portrayer of fantastic dwarfs, giants, elves, fairies, and gnomes, of sea serpents and water nymphs, of humanized animals and trees, was partially due to his release from the constraining bonds of newspaper reporting. Whatever the cause, this imaginative outpouring led to a highly lucrative career in book illustration, with such early successes as *Rip Van Winkle, Peter Pan,* and *Alice in Wonderland.*

Arthur Rackham created a world that combines the natural with the make-believe. His trees, clutching at the soil with their characteristically gnarled roots, often stretching down to a river of water, his rocks and bubbling brooks, his fields and flying birds often have an air of realistic repose, not unlike that of a John Constable landscape. If we look a little closer, however, down among the tree roots, or in the hollow of a hill, we may find a myriad of little creatures, gnomelike, with pointed noses, each often clothed in proper working attire and industriously pursuing his appointed occupation. In *The Little People's Market,* for example, this "wee world" is a flourishing social gathering, with an accordian-playing frog, gnome-sized baskets of fruit and eggs, bandana-headed merchants and a cache of wee tea ware. Yet some very real chipmunks are gazing at the goings-on! In *By the Way,* a row of red toadstools is transformed into a row of red-hatted elves and it's just possible, if we look again, we will see them transformed back into the row of red toadstools!

Rackham's work is marked by an extremely wide range of creativity—from the grotesque to the fanciful to the romantically realistic. His *Sea Serpent* is a masterpiece of scaly horror. Beady-eyed and slithering, it reminds one of the "slimy things" in Coleridge's "The Rime of the Ancient Mariner." His illustration for *The Frog Prince* is regal: columns of giant trees suggest a palace, and a golden-haired princess awes the minuscule and subservient little frog. *The Broad Walk* captures the romantic beauty of Kensington Gardens; its well-dressed ladies, running children, and Renoir-like little girls are a pleasant interlude in the Rackham imagery.

It is interesting to note that many of Rackham's gnomes, with their spectacles, pointed noses, and balding heads, look quite like him. Did the artist become so enmeshed in his imaginary world that he was part of t? Or, was he the well-adjusted person who could step back and readily poke fun at himself? Evidence supports the latter—it is said that his character had no faults; that he was practical, methodical, and well-loved. Indeed, he ministered to the need of children for fairies, but he also ministered to the need of adults.

Considered by many to be the most eminent illustrator of his day, Arthur Rackham achieved fame by illustrating the works of other men. Here, in large part, are his own ideas, his own interpretations of well-known themes of literature and his own flights of fancy. Although many may have been commissioned originally as illustrations for books, they are presented in this collection as a representation of the artist himself.

ELIZABETH CONGDON KOVANEN

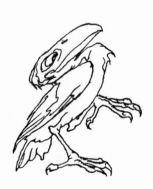

PICTURES

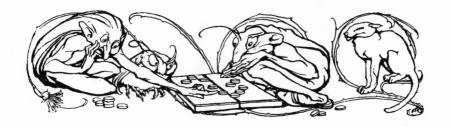

I OF·THE LITTLE PEOPLE

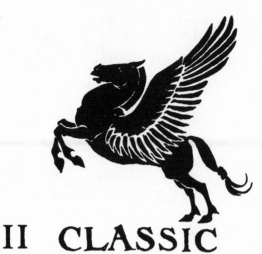

II CLASSIC

10 DANAË

Danaë was the daughter of the king of Argos, Acrisius. An oracle had foretold that she would one day give birth to a son, who would kill her father. So Acrisius for safety's sake shut her up in a tower, where, nevertheless, she was visited by Zeus in a shower of gold and became the mother of Perseus. Acrisius put the mother and child into a chest and exposed them on the sea. But the chest drifted ashore on the island of Seriphos, Danaë and her child were saved and Perseus lived to fulfil the oracle's prophecy.

11 THE DRAGON OF THE HESPERIDES

12 DRYAD

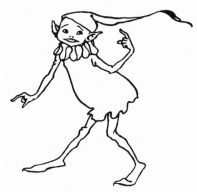

III SOME FAIRY TALES

13 JACK THE GIANT KILLER

In the course of his adventures, Jack sleeps at
the house of a monstrous Welsh giant with two
heads. In the morning he has breakfast with
the giant. Each has a bowl containing four
gallons of hasty pudding. "One would have
thought that the greater portion of so extrava-
gant an allowance would have been declined by
our hero, but he was unwilling the giant should
imagine his incapability to eat it, and accordingly
placed a large leather bag under his loose coat in
such a position that he could convey the pudding
into it without the deception being perceived.
Breakfast at length being finished, Jack excited
the giant's curiosity by offering to show him an
extraordinary sleight of hand ; so taking a knife,
he ripped the leather bag, and out, of course,
descended on the ground all the hasty pudding.
The giant had not the slightest suspicion of the
trick, veritably believing the pudding came from
its natural receptacle, and having the same
antipathy to being beaten, exclaimed in true
Welsh, 'Odds splutters, hur can do that trick
hurself.' The sequel may be readily guessed.
The monster took the knife, and thinking to
follow Jack's example with impunity, killed
himself on the spot."

14 JACK AND THE BEAN STALK

Jack clambers down the beanstalk and chops it through with his axe ; and the giant who is descending after him falls to the earth and is killed.

15 PUSS IN BOOTS

Puss in Boots was the sole possession of a poor youth. The cat, however, manages by a succession of clever tricks to make his master's fortune. He gains for him the fine castle and vast estates that belonged to an ogre by the same device that Loge used to get the Ring of the Niblungs from Alberich. He calls at the castle and, by pretending to doubt the ogre's magic powers, he induces him to change himself first into a lion and then into a mouse, whereupon he falls upon him and eats him up.

Perrault.

16 ADRIFT

"I will put on my new red shoes," she said one morning, "those which Kay has not seen, and then I will go down to the river and ask it about him."

It was quite early ; little Gerda kissed her old grandmother, who was asleep, put on the red shoes, and went out quite alone through the town gate towards the river.

" Is it true that you have taken my little playmate ? I will make you a present of my red shoes if you will give him back to me."

And she thought the waves nodded to her so strangely ; she then took her red shoes, the most precious she had, and threw them both out into the river, but they fell close to the bank and the little billows soon carried them ashore to her ; it seemed as if the river would not take the dearest treasure she had because it could not give back little Kay to her ; but then she thought she had not thrown the shoes out far enough, and so she climbed into a boat which was lying among the rushes, and went right to the farthest end of it and threw the shoes into the water ; but the boat was not fastened, and its motion as she got into it sent it adrift from the bank. As soon as she noticed this she hastened to get out of the boat, but before she could jump ashore it was an arm's length from the bank, and it drifted rapidly down the river.

The Snow Queen.
Andersen.

17 THE FROG PRINCE

The youngest daughter of the King loses her golden ball in a well in the forest where she has been playing. A frog hears her crying and bargains with her before he fetches back her ball. He will not accept her offer of her pretty dresses, or her pearls or diamonds, or even of her golden crown, but makes her promise that she will be fond of him and let him be her playmate, sit by her at table, eat out of her plate, drink out of her cup and sleep in her little bed—" if you will promise all this," he says, " I will dive down and bring you back your golden ball." Of course she agrees, thinking she may safely promise a frog anything he asks no matter how absurd it is. The frog brings back her ball, and the Princess has to keep all her promises much to her chagrin. But all ends happily. The frog proves to be a bewitched Prince, is restored to his natural form, and marries the Princess.

Grimm.

18 SANTA CLAUS

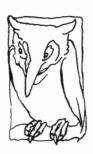

IV

SOME · CHILDREN ·

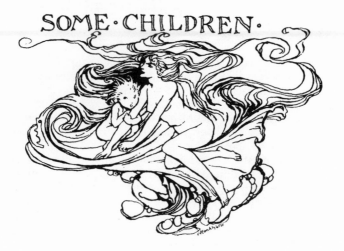

"In the Broad Walk, you meet all the people who are worth knowing."

Peter Pan in Kensington Gardens.

J. M. Barrie.

V

GROTESQUE

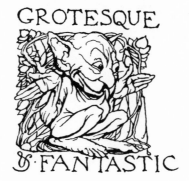

& FANTASTIC

"He maketh the deep to boil like a pot . . . . . .
He maketh a path to shine after him ; one would
think the deep to be hoary."

VI   VARIOUS

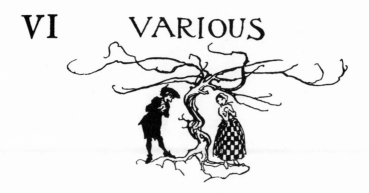

34   CUPID'S ALLEY

" O, Love's but a dance,
Where Time plays the fiddle!
See the couples advance,—
O, Love's but a dance!
A whisper, a glance,—
' Shall we twirl down the middle?'
O, Love's but a dance,
Where Time plays the fiddle!

      *   *   *

"Strange Dance! 'Tis free to Rank and Rags;
  Here no distinction flatters,
Here riches shakes its money-bags,
  And Poverty its tatters;
Church, Army, Navy, Physic, Law;—
  Maid, Mistress, Master, Valet;
Long locks, grey hairs, bald heads, and a',—
  They bob—in ' Cupid's Alley.'"

Austin Dobson.

The picture is in the National Gallery of British Art.

35   BASTINADO

36   THE FAIRY WIFE

" In a mild and steady light, which came from no
illumination of moon or stars, but seemed to be
interfused with the air, in the strong, warm wind
which wrapped the fell-top upon a sward of bent
grass which ran toward the tarn and ended in

swept reeds, he saw six young women dancing in a ring. Not to any music that he could hear did they move, nor was the rhythm of their movement either ordered or wild. It was not formal dancing, and it was not at all a Bacchic rout: rather they flitted hither and thither on the turf, now touching hands, now straining heads to one another, crossing, meeting, parting, winding about and about with the purposeless and untirable frivolity of moths. They seemed neither happy nor unhappy, they made no sound ; it looked to the lad as if they had been so drifting from the beginning, and would so drift to the end of things temporal.

*   *   *   *

" . . . . then, circling round him, they swept him forward on the wind, past Silent Water, over the Edge, out on to the fells, on and on and on, and never stopped till they had reached Knapp Forest, that dreadful place.

"There, in the hushed aisles and glades, they played with this new found creature—played with him, fought for him, and would have loved him if he had been minded for such adventuring.

*   *   *   *

"Andrew King, like young Tamlane, might have sojourned with them for ever and a day but for one thing. He saw by chance a seventh maiden—a white-faced, woebegone, horror-struck Seventh Sister, blenched and frozen under a great beech. She may have been there throughout his commerce with the rest, or she may have been revealed to him in a flash then and there. So as it was, he saw her suddenly, and thereafter saw no other at all. She held his eyes waking ; he left his playmates and went to her, where she crouched."

Maurice Hewlett.

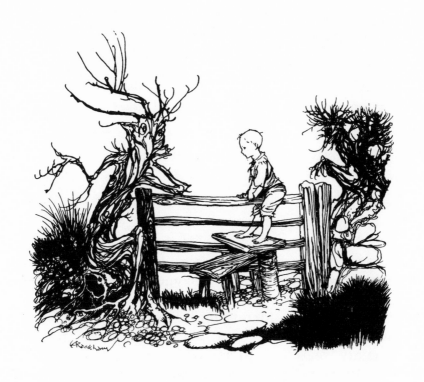

INTRODUCTION

HE owner of this book, as he turns its pages and criticises the drawings, will very likely pronounce No. 21, *The Broad Walk, Kensington Gardens,* to be the least imaginative of all, and even wonder how it came to be included amid so much finely imaginative work. Well, without consulting Mr. Rackham I will give a guess (which, when you are concerned with fantasy, is often more useful than knowing), and if my guess be right, this No. 21 is a very significant drawing indeed. All I *know* of it is what Mr. Rackham's modesty deigns to tell me: that it originally appeared in *The Century Magazine,* when it accompanied—but did not profess to illustrate—an article by Lady St. Helier on "The

Training of Children."* I have not read that article, but the artist might well have meant to illustrate its abhorrent title. You observe that by the rails of the Broad Walk he actually allows "grown-ups" to stalk unchecked, like respectability at Chicago: and as for the three well-dressed little girls standing correctly by hoops which they forbear to trundle—we have the best authority for saying that they ought not to be in the Broad Walk at all. Their place is obviously in the contiguous "Figs."

> The Gardens are a tremendous big place, with millions and hundreds of trees; and first you come to the Figs, but you scorn to loiter there, for the Figs is the resort of superior little persons, who are forbidden to mix with the commonalty, and is so named, according to legend, because they dress in full fig. These dainty ones are themselves contemptuously called Figs. . . . Occasionally a rebel Fig climbs over the fence into the world. . . .

—which is the Broad Walk. So says Sir James Barrie, and what he does not know about Kensington Gardens is notoriously not worth knowing. For the key of the picture, then, you are to look down at the lower left-hand corner, at the three small children running. There is no stupid "training" in these three: and if you ask whither they run, the more obvious answer is, for the Hump ("which is the part of the Broad Walk where all the big races are run") or the Round Pond ("where you can't be good all the time, however much you try"); but the truer one, that they chase those childish visions with which their interpreter, the

*I hasten to add in a footnote that this is one of the very few drawings that have appeared elsewhere.

author of *Peter Pan*—himself interpreted and helped by a draughtsman of imagination—has peopled the Gardens for us. Now this second interpreter, this helper, is Mr. Arthur Rackham.

At Lancaster Gate, past which the omnibuses ply between Shepherd's Bush and the Marble Arch (poetical names), there stands a house overlooking, across that wide river of traffic, the delectable haunts of Peter Pan; and in that house the author of Peter Pan's being first informed me (for proof, leading me to a painted panel over the fireplace) that he had really and truly found an artist to understand his mystery. (He put it more modestly, but that is what he meant.) I took leave to be incredulous; but in due course there appeared the now famous edition of the book, with Mr. Rackham's drawings, and I recanted.

When Wordsworth told our grandfathers or great-grandfathers that

Heaven lies about us in our infancy,

he was reviving what had been a favourite fancy with the old seventeenth-century writers, Henry Vaughan, Thomas Traherne, John Earle. "The elder he grows," says Earle concerning a Child in his *Microcosmography*, "he is a stair lower from God; and, like his first father, much worse in his breeches . . . Could he put off his body with his little coat, he had got eternity without a burden, and exchanged but one heaven for another." "Certainly Adam in Paradise had not more sweet and curious apprehensions of the world than I when I was a child," writes Traherne in his *Centuries of Meditations*.

I was a little stranger which at my entrance into the world was saluted and surrounded with innumerable joys. My knowledge was divine. I knew by intuition those things which, since my Apostasy, I collected again by the highest reason . . . I knew nothing of sickness or death or rents or exaction, either for tribute or bread. In the absence of these I was entertained like an Angel with the works of God in their splendour and glory. I saw all in the peace of Eden . . . The corn was orient and immortal wheat, which never should be reaped nor was ever sown. . . . The dust and stones of the street were as precious as gold. The gates were at first the end of the world. The green trees, when I saw them first through one of the gates, transported and ravished me; their sweetness and unusual beauty made my heart to leap and almost mad with ecstasy . . . Boys and girls, tumbling in the streets and playing, were moving jewels. I knew not that they were born or should die: but all things abided eternally as they were in their proper places. . . . The city seemed to stand in Eden, or to be built in Heaven. The streets were mine, the temple was mine, the people were mine, their clothes and gold and silver were mine, as much as their sparkling eyes, fair skins and ruddy faces. The skies were mine and so were the sun and moon and stars, and all the World was mine; and I the only spectator and enjoyer of it. . . . So that with much ado I was corrupted and made to learn the dirty devices of this world. Which now I unlearn, and become as it were a little child again that I may enter into the Kingdom of God.

All the critics, again, send us harking back from Wordsworth's great Ode, to compare it with Vaughan's exquisite *Retreat:*—

> Happy those early days when I
> Shined in my Angel-infancy! . . .
> When yet I had not walk'd above
> A mile or two from my first Love,
> And looking back, at that short space,

Could see a glimpse of His bright face:
When on some gilded cloud or flower
My gazing soul would dwell an hour,
And in those weaker glories spy
Some shadows of Eternity . . .

But Wordsworth did more than merely revive a lovely fancy out of the dust of eighteenth-century rationalism. He did, up to a point, about the best thing a poet can do; he told men something they all knew concerning themselves, but had grown shy of confessing. [As George Eliot wrote of him, "I never before met with so many of my own feelings expressed just as I should like them."] And he told it in such a way that, as men looked in one another's faces and read confession, this inveterate shame fell from them. "Hullo!" said Smith in effect, "here are Brown and Jones guilty of recollections just as frantic as those I have been hiding under my tall hat! Let us all own up."

Rome, however, was not built in a day: and shy, conventional men and women, after a shock, must be given a rest and a pause or two before they shed all their humbug. It was a great feat of Wordsworth's to force out of our great-grandfathers an admission that they had been even *celestially* minded in their infancy. That they had been at once *celestially and ludicrously* minded was more than they could be expected to allow. Nor, in truth, was Wordsworth the man to compel them, for here his vision extended no farther than theirs. He had scarcely any sense of the ludicrous, and certainly no happy familiar understanding of it: while in philosophy (if the truth must be told) he was something of an amateur and very much of the maiden aunt. Now in dealing with childish things, as in dealing with love or things divine, there are two stages of initiation; of which the first, which is all awe and seriousness, has a knack of being taken for the higher; whereas it is in truth rawer and more elementary than the insight which, having taught you to adore, permits you also to smile; as a good husband may (because the understanding is perfect) "chaff" his wife and at the same time love her more deeply than he ever did in the merely reverential days of court-ship.

In truth Heaven does lie about us in our infancy (let us note in passing, but to scorn it, the *paranomasia* of the wretched cynic who added "and we return the compliment during the rest of our lives"). But the child's Heaven, like the child's earth, is a mixture of the mysterious and the definite, the practical and the absurd. The child himself, set between the mysterious and the absurd, is all the while severely practical. He wants to know how creation was managed; he wants (in the words of that half-forgotten American book, *Helen's Babies)* to see the wheels go round; he wants to know who made the trees, ships, life-guards-men, the sea, bathing machines, porridge, jam, uncles and aunts—of trees and jam (for example) *how*—and of uncles and aunts (for example) *why?* He takes an amazing interest in God as the inventor and patentee of such things. "Did he make the elephant, Mummy?" "Yes, dear." "And the flea?" "Yes, dear." "Niggling little job, that." And why should anyone omnipotently free to make a mud-pie have made Uncle John instead?

Above all, seeing that "the world is so full of a number

of things"—having grown tired, for example, of trying to count the buttercups in the near meadow—he declines the idea of a single Demiurge turning out all these marvels from one great lonely laboratory. For that, besides being unthinkable, is not at all how things happen in real life, down in the village, where, although that wonderful fellow the blacksmith might at first sight seem, like Habakkuk, capable of anything—such marvels issue from his forge— yet Sam the cobbler measures you for your shoes, and old Eppett mends the gates, and Blind Harry weaves the baskets. No, the Demiurge cannot possibly find time for it all. He *must* employ hosts of small unseen workmen. As Mr. Thorley says of these same buttercups—

> There *must* be fairy miners—

See them going to their work, in No. 3.

> There *must* be fairy miners
>   Just underneath the mould,
> Such wondrous quaint designers,
>   Who live in caves of gold.
>
> They take the shining metals,
>   And beat them into shreds;
> And mould them into petals
>   To make the flowers' heads . . .
>
> And still a tiny fan turns
>   Above a forge of gold—

So far the child. The reflective man finishes the stanza:

> To keep with fairy lanterns
>   The world from growing old.

Therefore, even if there were no such beings as fairies,

25

the children would have to invent them—pixies, nixies, gnomes, goblins, elves, kobbolds, and the rest—to account for the marvels that are happening all the while, but especially while we sleep. How else can we explain toadstools, for instance?

To this instant, constant, intellectual need of childhood no one in our day has ministered so bountifully or so whole-heartedly as Mr. Rackham; and the drawings in this book—as they were not invented to order, to serve some other fellow's invention—prove that he does his spiriting *con amore* and with belief in it. A few, to be sure, play with familiar stories, *Jack the Giant-Killer, Jack and the Beanstalk, Puss in Boots.* But turn back a few pages and pause at No. 5, which he calls simply *By the Way.* A princess, wandering down a country road, stops to pass the time of day with some toadstools. That is all. There is no story: or, rather, there must be a story, only you have to make it up for yourself. Something sang in Mr. Rackham's head—possibly Meredith's "Let not your fair princess stray"—and the fancy grew out of it. But note how definitely he gives us what is magical, the change of the toadstools into elves; and contrariwise with what a delicate sense of mystery he treats what is ordinary—how the ploughed furrows converge towards the cottage on the brow of the hill, drawing us on to surmise a land of greater marvels beyond the horizon, "over the hills and far away," beneath the sunset into which the birds are homing. (Compare with this the landscape in *Shades of Evening,* No. 32.) Or take No. 6, *The Little People's Market*—not at all the Goblin Market of Miss Christina Rossetti's poem, but a chatty sociable market among the little folk themselves. Who that has been a child has not longed to surprise some such jolly goings-on, say in the depths of a disused rabbit-warren by the base of an old tree?

Mr. Rackham has a wonderful sense of trees and their mystery; nor need I go to learned works, such as Mr. Frazer's *Golden Bough,* to prove what everybody knows, that to suggest meditation or stir the imagination in human beings there is nothing comparable with an old tree, especially if it reach down its roots, half-exposed, towards running water. (Observe the tree in No. 1, *The Magic Cup;* and again the trees in Nos. 22, *The Green Dragon,* and 4, *Goblin Thieves,* for different treatments of this theme.) If you remember, it was by such a tree that the youthful dreamer in Gray's Elegy fed his wayward fancies:

> There at the foot of yonder nodding beech,
>   That wreathes its old fantastic roots so high,
> His listless length at noontide would he stretch
>   And pore upon the brook that bubbles by.

As it was by such a tree (an oak, this time) that the melancholy Jaques meditated:

> as he lay along
> Under an oak whose antique root peeps out,
> Upon the brook that brawls along the world.

(I passed that very tree the other day, as I paddled in a canoe down Shakespeare's Avon, through the Forest of Arden, which is Stoneleigh Park, in Arden of Warwickshire.)

For imaginative men, since the beginning of the world, each tree conceals a spirit, as Ariel was held in the cloven pine; nor can you pull up one of these roots but something almost human cries out at the laceration, as Polydorus screamed from the root of the cornel when Æneas tugged at it. In drawing after drawing within these covers you may detect this "tree-spirit" striving to liberate or to declare itself; and it takes human form exquisitely (to my thinking) in Nos. 36, *The Fairy Wife,* and 12, *A Dryad.*

But in these Mr. Rackham has travelled far away from the children, to whom let us recur for a moment before we follow his more elderly, maybe more poetical, inventions. A rat-hole in a river bank, or a rabbit-hole by the roots of a secular beech—"dull must he be of soul who could pass by" either of these as a child without peopling them in imagination.

> A rat-hole by the river's brim
> Only a rat-hole was to him—

If such blindness ever afflicted boy or girl in my benighted generation, how can it in this, for which Mr. Kenneth Grahame has written *The Wind in the Willows,* a book all concerned with these fascinating lairs? (I remember a school-fellow nudging me once in church with a "Now then, shout!" when the choir reached the verse "The high hills are a refuge for the wild goats; *and so are the stony rocks for the conies";* and still in mature years I feel in my ribs that ghostly elbow (long since, alas! a bone in the grave) when some poor fellow comes up arraigned before his fellow-sinners for the offence of trespassing in pursuit of conies. [1 and 2, William IV., c. 32. "If any person whatsoever shall commit any trespass by entering or being in the day-time upon any land in search or pursuit of game, or of woodcocks, snipes, quails, landrails or conies"—Penalty not exceeding £2 and costs.] But, though rabbit-holes are the most obviously tempting things in Nature, you never know where a child's imagination will go exploring. One will be content with no less than piracy on the high seas, "keel-hauling," walking the plank; another with no less than the warfare of Red Indians, and a waistband hung with bleeding scalps; while a third (as Mr. Grahame again has taught us) will haunt Pall Mall, S.W. in fancy, and suppose himself, with an awed surmise, a full-blooded member of the Athenæum or of the Army and Navy Club.

I doubt, if Mr. Rackham has ever illustrated such an achievement as that; yet feel sure that he would do it justice, so whole-heartedly he will be a child and play with any child in its mood. *Quicquid agunt pueri*. . . . Someone, criticising him adversely the other day (as we shall none of us escape censure), suggested that "it was not very funny, after all, to draw people with long noses." To this I answer, "Not very funny in our eyes, perhaps—though quite a large number of grown-ups have laughed at Cyrano de Bergerac; but very funny indeed, or at any rate highly interesting, to the unsophisticated child. *Ah! quel drôle de nez!* In the growth and removal of a long nose consists all the plot of Madame Leprince de Beaumont's *Le Prince Désir,* a little classic which Andrew Lang thought worthy of a place in *The Blue Fairy Book,* his first and best. And were we not all thrilled, once on a time, by the elongation of Alice's neck, as portrayed by Tenniel in *Alice in Wonderland?* You will be suggesting next that Bluebeard might as well be Greybeard!" . . . No, children do not look for fun in these abnormalities, but take them rather with a deep seriousness; and in his pawky seriousness lies something of Mr. Rackham's secret as an illustrator of fairyland. Consider it in No. 30, *Mother Goose.* We know, and Mr. Rackham knows, that when the snow falls it is shed by the old lady aloft plucking geese. But observe the effect of this phenomenon upon the good folk of Paisley, who pace about preoccupied with earth and their own affairs, having no eyes for the clouds or what lies beyond. (I call the town Paisley, not because I have ever been there to recognise it, but one of the ladies is taking the air in a Paisley shawl, and anyhow I don't know where else it is likely to be.)

No. 36, *The Fairy Wife* (a most poetical thing to my mind), was first drawn for a little story by Mr. Maurice Hewlett—a gem afterwards reset and since famous as *Pan and the Young Shepherd.* No. 19, *Marjorie and Margaret,* is a portrait study, more or less. No. 34, *Cupid's Alley,* was inspired by Mr. Austin Dobson's well-known poem. This drawing hangs in the Tate Gallery.

Nos. 1, 3, 6, 9, 28 and 30 began as "Langham Sketches"; Nos. 9 and 28 being "Langham Sketches" virtually untouched. Now for the reader ignorant—as was I, a while ago—what a "Langham Sketch" may be, let the following explanation be provided: The "Langham Sketch Club"—adorned in its time, which is not yet over, by a large number of very respectable draughtsmen and by some very famous ones, such as Fred Walker and Charles Keene—is a gathering of artists who meet on Friday evenings; when from seven to nine o'clock all work on a given subject. At nine there is a "show-up"; that is, the resulting sketches are placed on a screen for exhibition and criticism. Meanwhile supper is preparing, and the rest of the evening takes that particular form of enjoyment as a more famous *soirée* took the form of a boiled leg of mutton and trimmings. From this report, which is all I can give, you may gather that at the Langham Sketch Club it is possible for men of social instincts but quiet minds to be happy enough and even happier than they know—*fortunati sua si bona norint.*

I trust, now, enough has been said to indicate that in this book Mr. Rackham, who has achieved much fame by illustrating the inventions of other men, has turned to illustrate himself; and the order of the drawings has been arranged so that you may follow, if you will, the liberation of his fancy. He begins by taking us to the land of the Little People, then in Nos. 10 to 17 (which is Grimm's *Frog Prince)* he keeps close to the well-known persons and stories of Faëry. Thenceforward for the most part we are among phantasies, playful or grotesque. In No. 23, for example, which he calls *Once upon a Time,* there seems to be a story but is none: he just brings together in a suggestive group nine or ten types without one or two of which no fairy tale is complete. All will recognise—besides the King and the Swineherd—the Goose-girl, the Knight, the Foundling and the little Princess. When we reach *Shades of Evening* and *The Fairy*

Wife, however, the book seems to lose something of definite purpose while it gains in beauty. We are now following the wayward visions that tease every true artist's mind, while he bends over the day's work. As one who has been doing the day's work in another form of art, and for more years than he cares to count, I wish it were possible for someone to make for me such a collection of fugitive impressions, hints of beauty, threads caught and followed (often tenaciously) only to be lost in the end; scraps of song; stories that after one bright apparition faded away into limbo. They would make one's best biography and, apart from the tale of work (such as it is) actually achieved, his only biography worth writing. Mr. Rackham has been more fortunate, and I congratulate him. But let the purchaser who, turning these pages, may happen to wish that they told a connected story, reflect that he may have hold of something better worth his money; the elusive dreams of an artist such as the goblin in Hans Andersen saw and adored for the moment as he peered down the chimney into the student's garret over the huckster's shop; the dreams of an artist who has taught English children in our time to see that

> All things by immortal power,
> Near or far,
> Hiddenly
> To each other linkèd are,
> That thou canst not stir a flower
> Without troubling of a star.

ARTHUR QUILLER-COUCH.

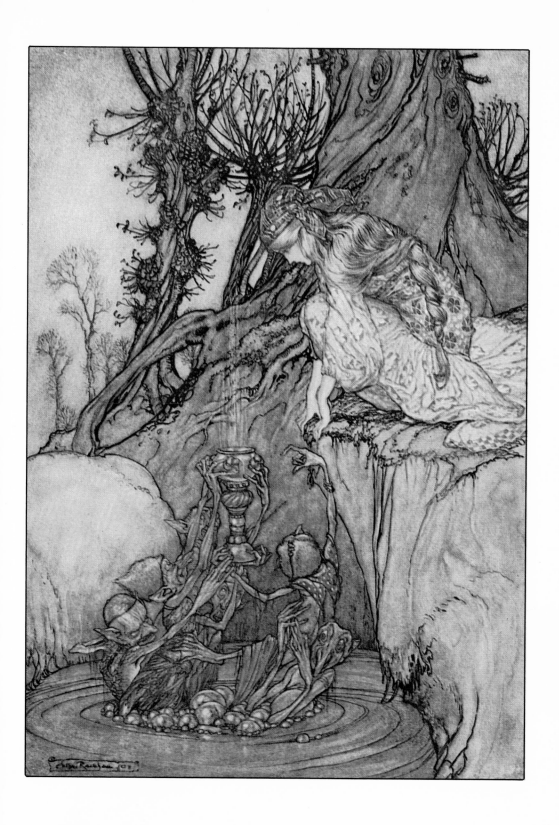

1   *The Magic Cup*

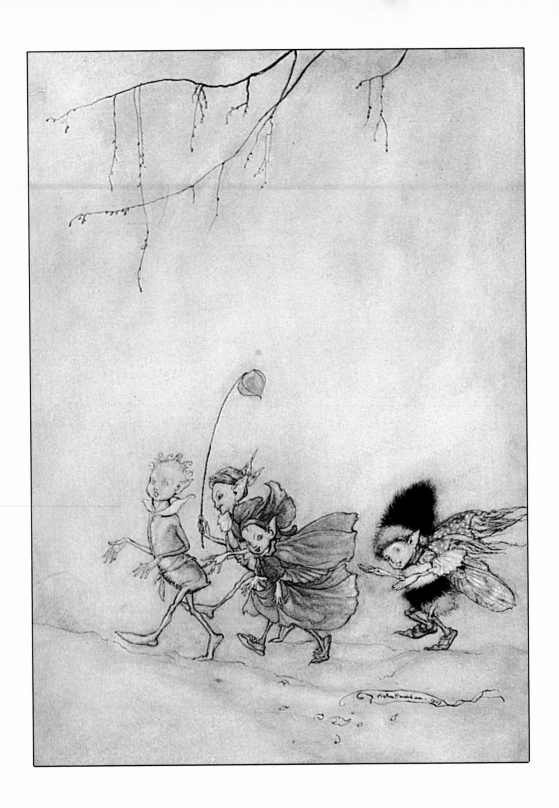

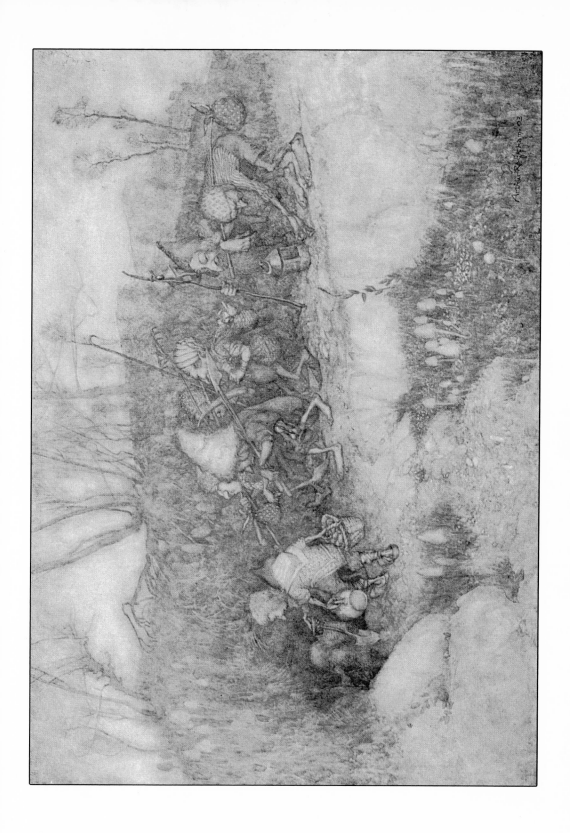

3   *Seekers for Treasure*

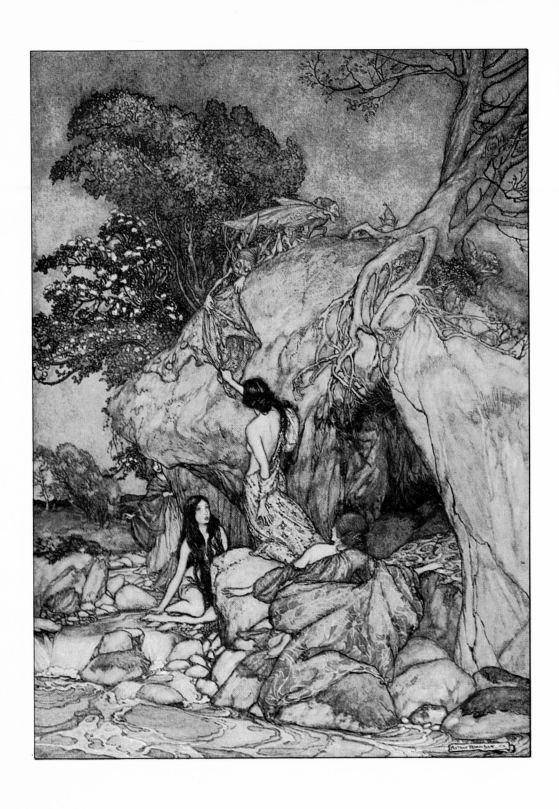

4   *Goblin Thieves*

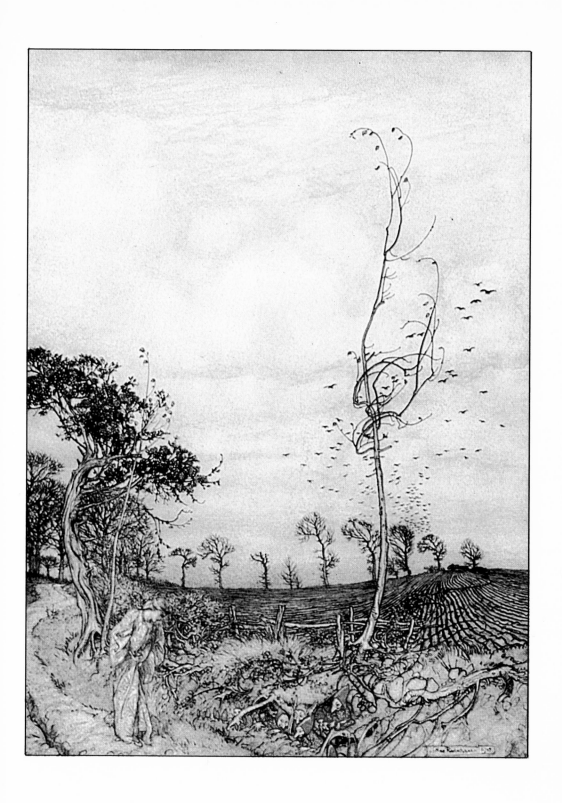

5   *By the Way*

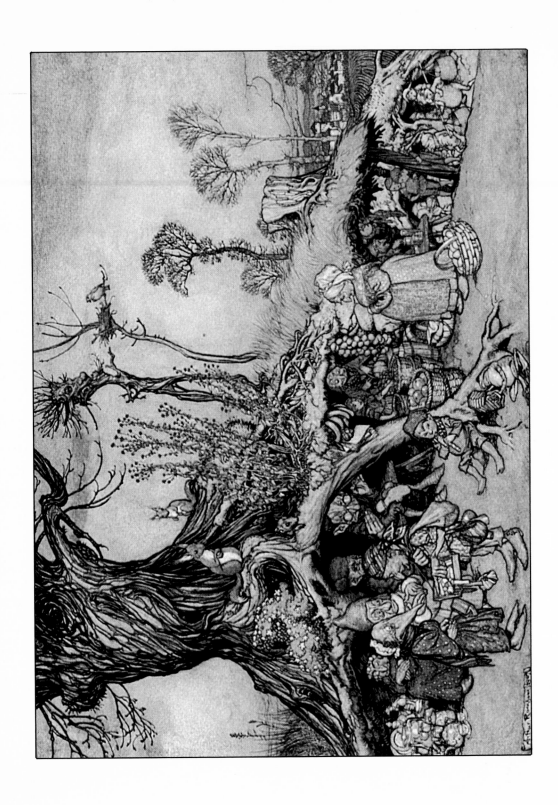

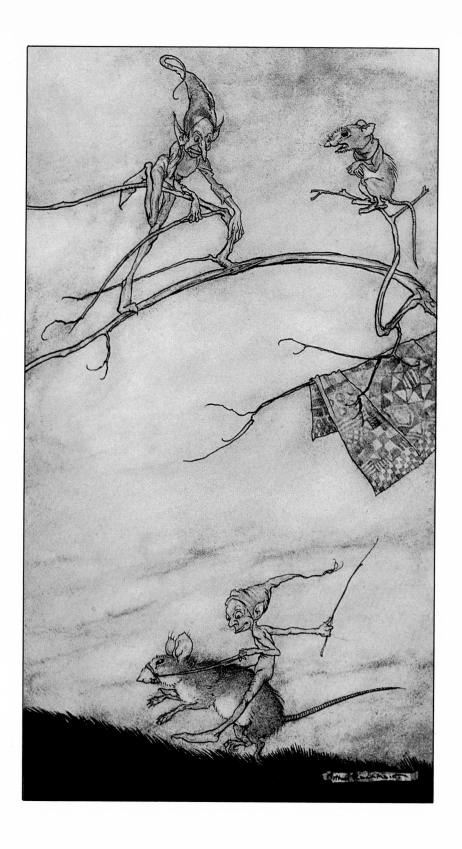

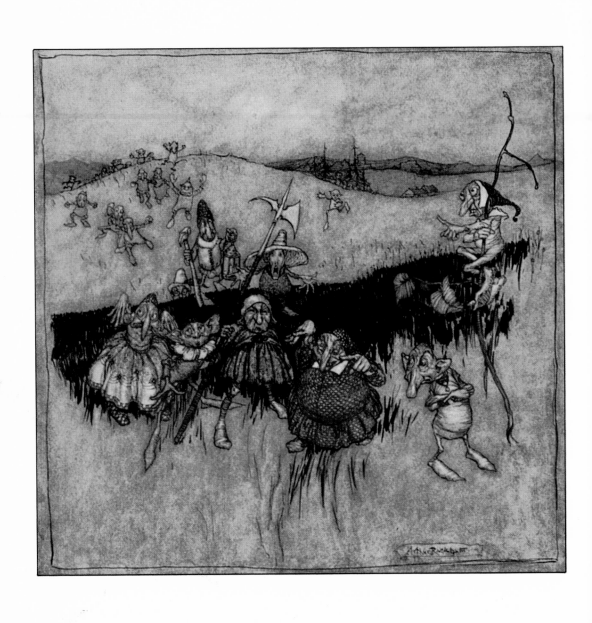

8   *Malice*

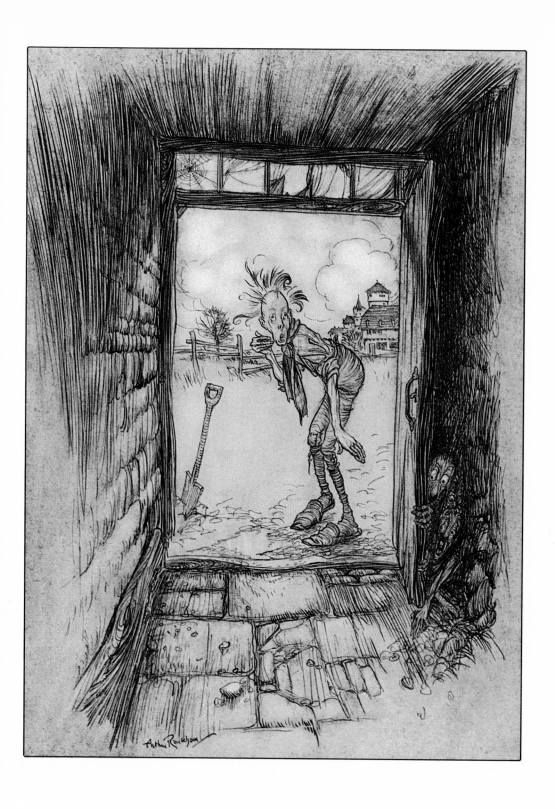

9   *The Man who was Terrified by Goblins*

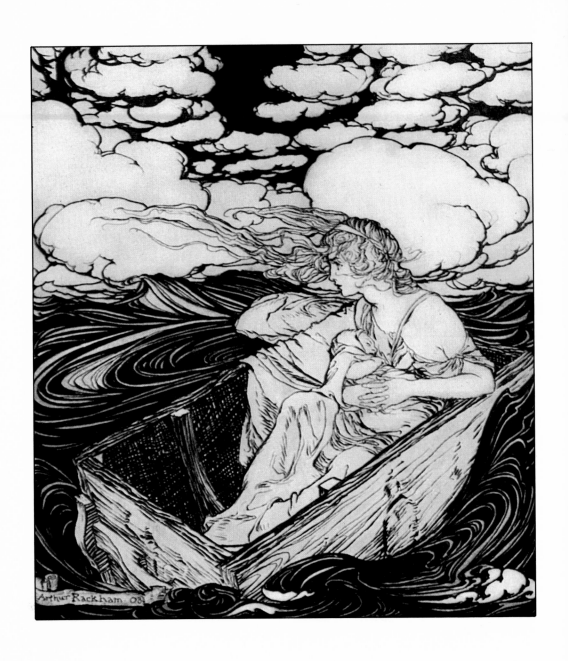

10   *Danaë*

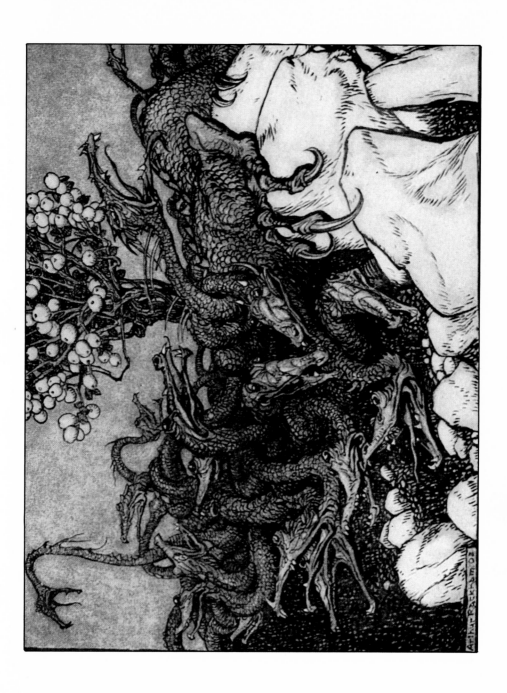

11   *The Dragon of the Hesperides*

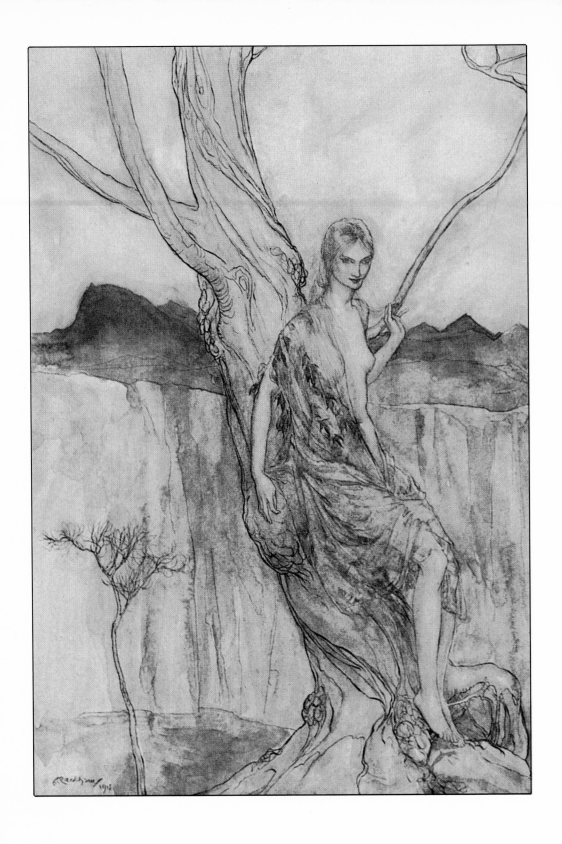

12   *Dryad*

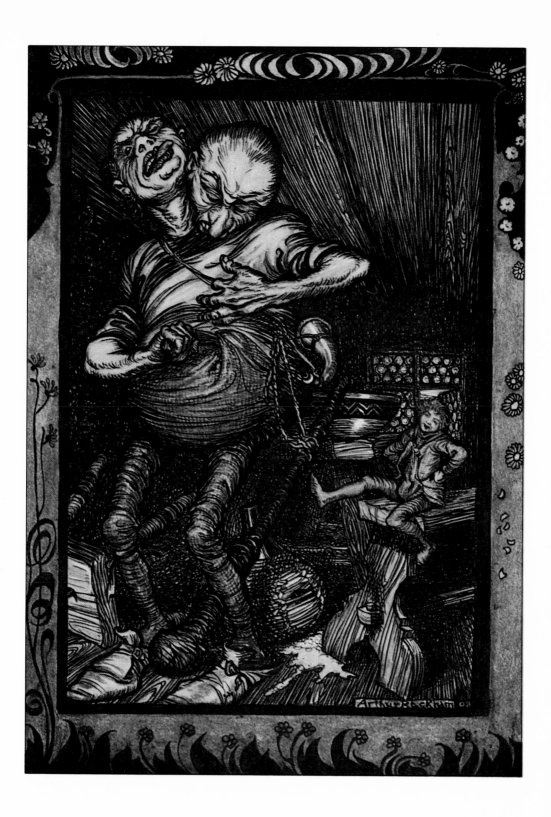

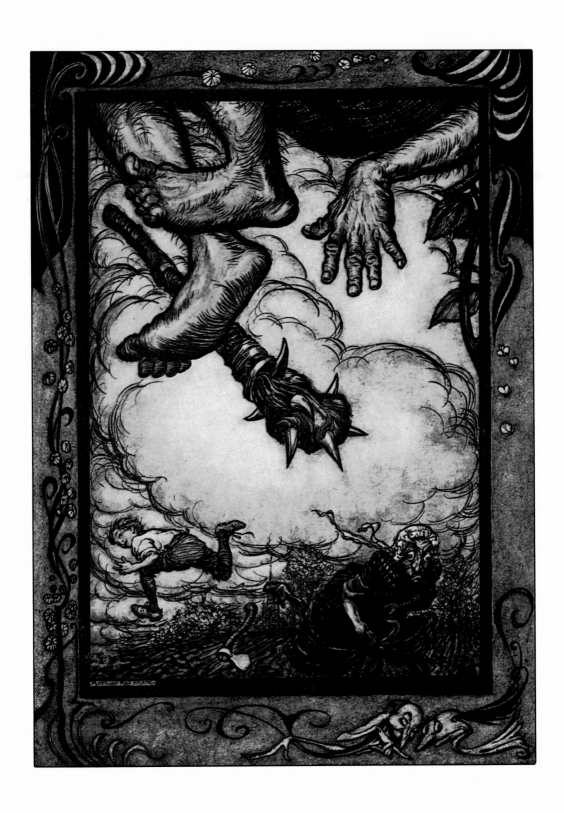

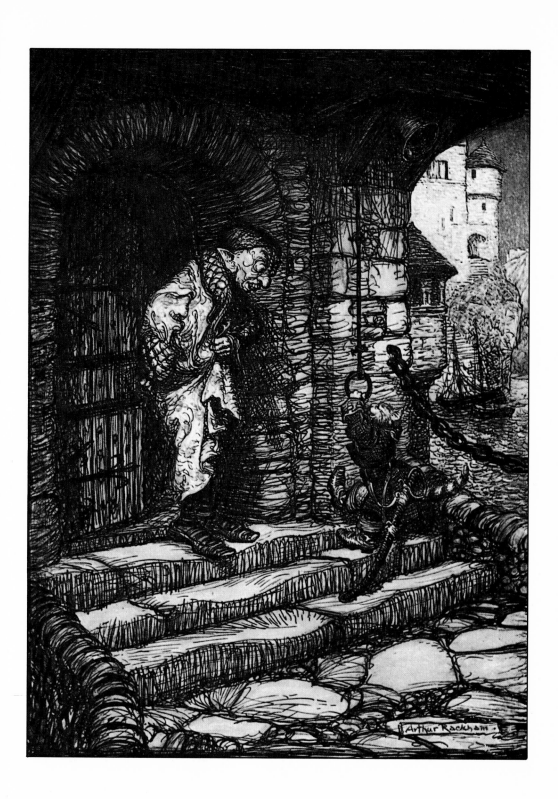

15   *Puss in Boots*

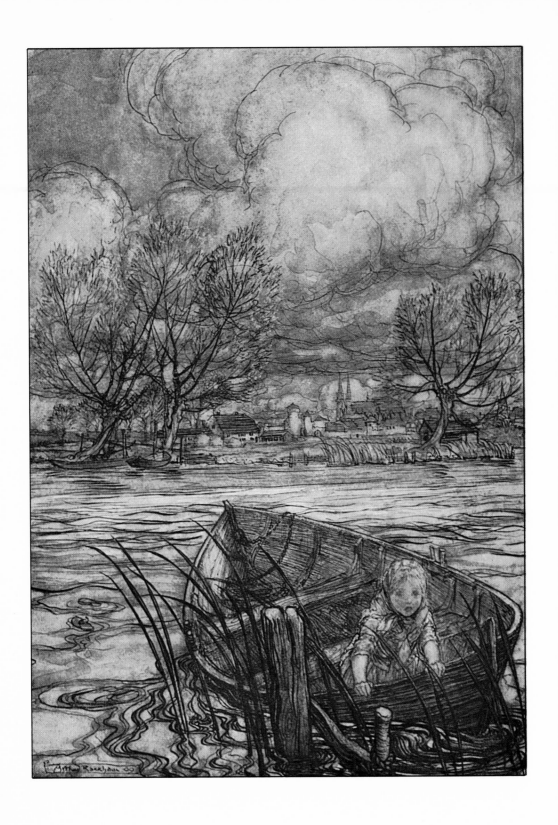

16   *Adrift*

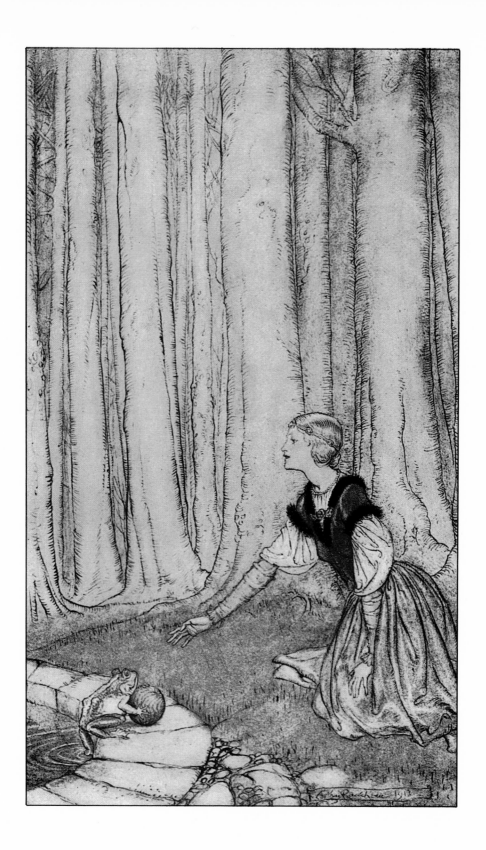

The Frog Prince

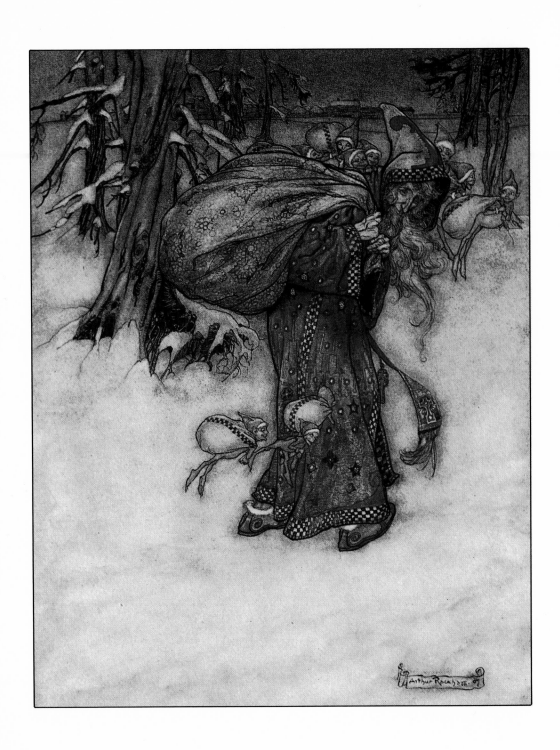

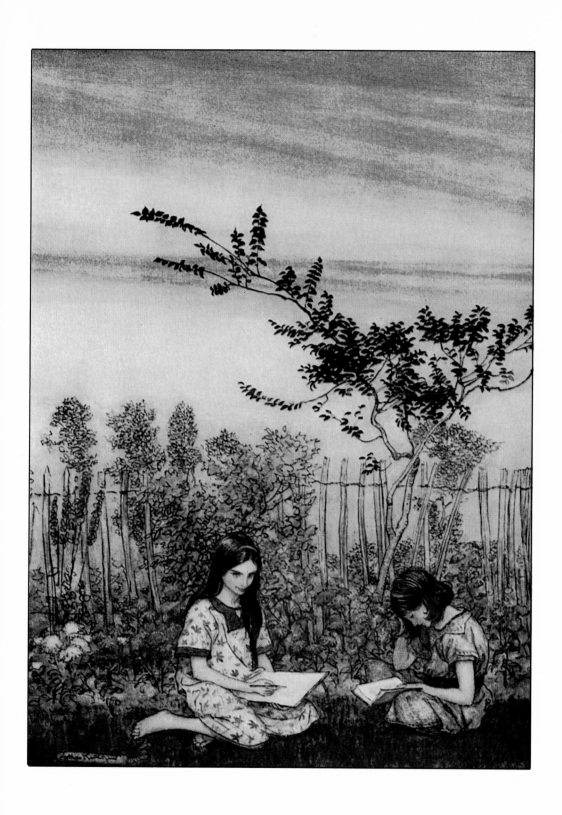

19   *Marjorie and Margaret*

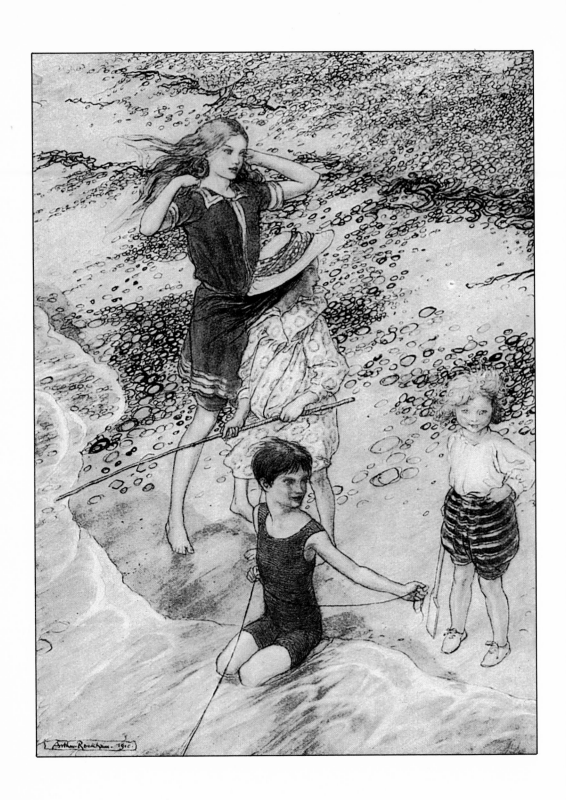

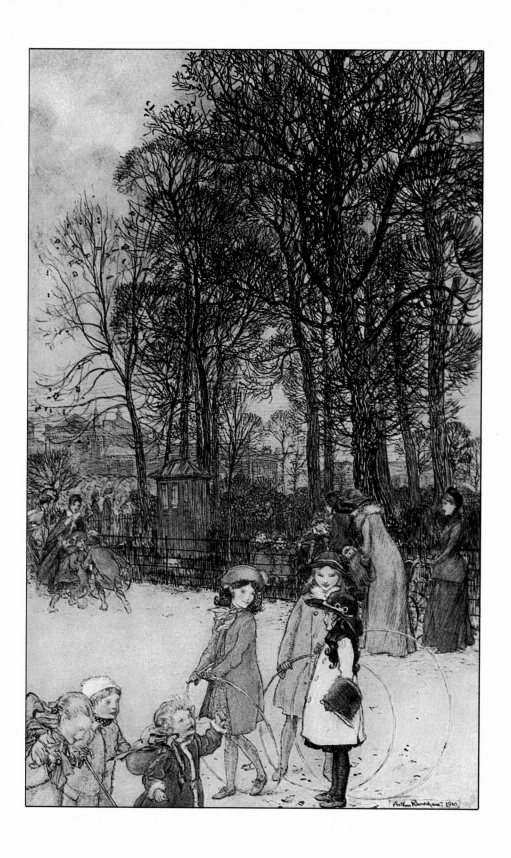

21   *The Broad Walk*

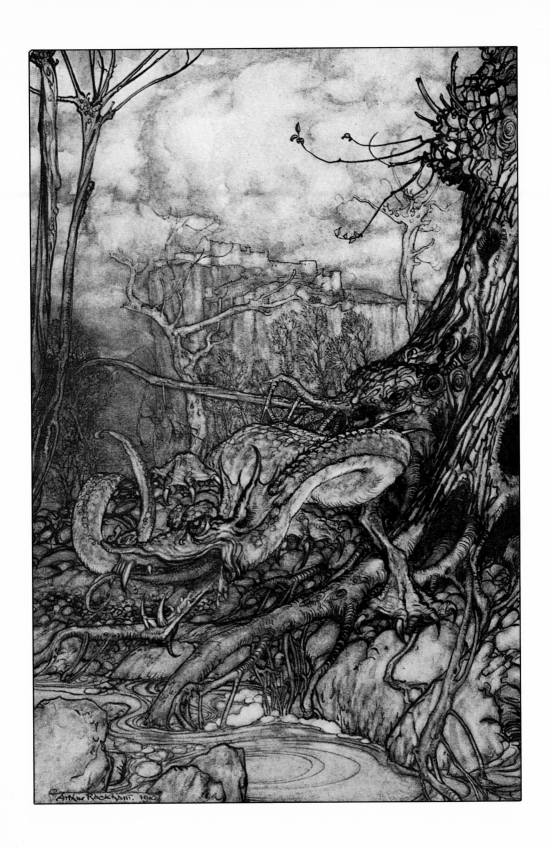

22   *The Green Dragon*

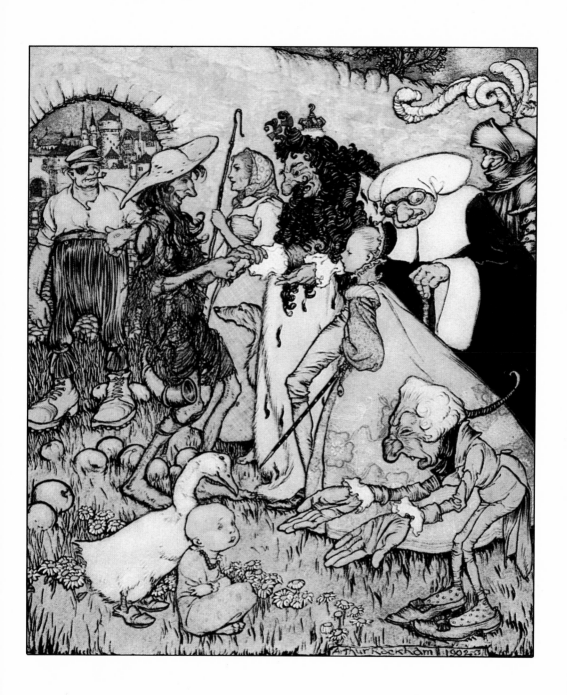

Once upon a Time

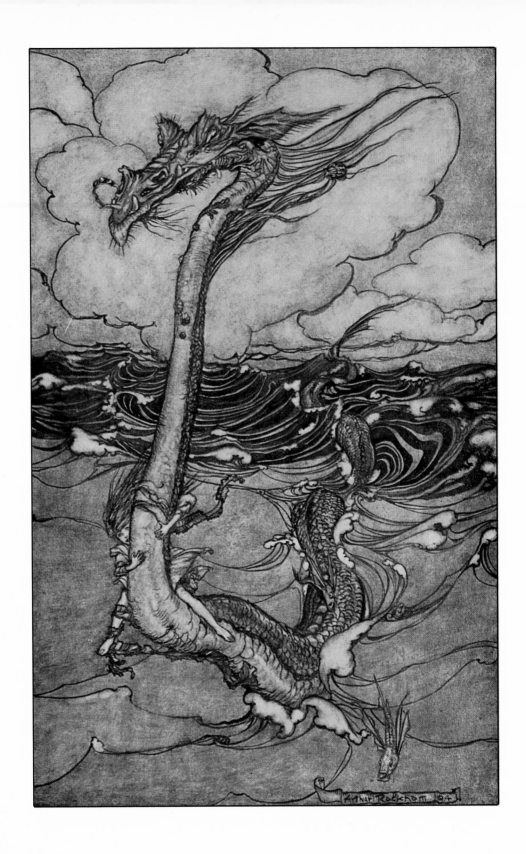

24   *The Sea Serpent*

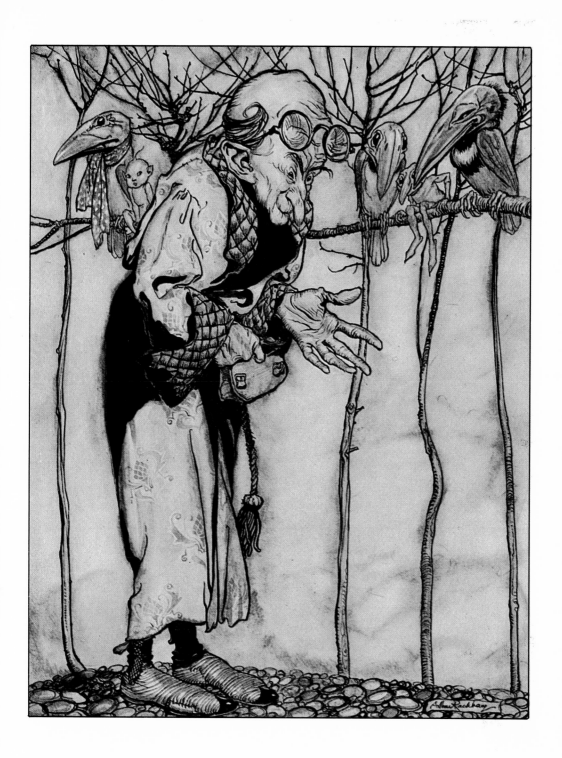

25   *The Wizard*

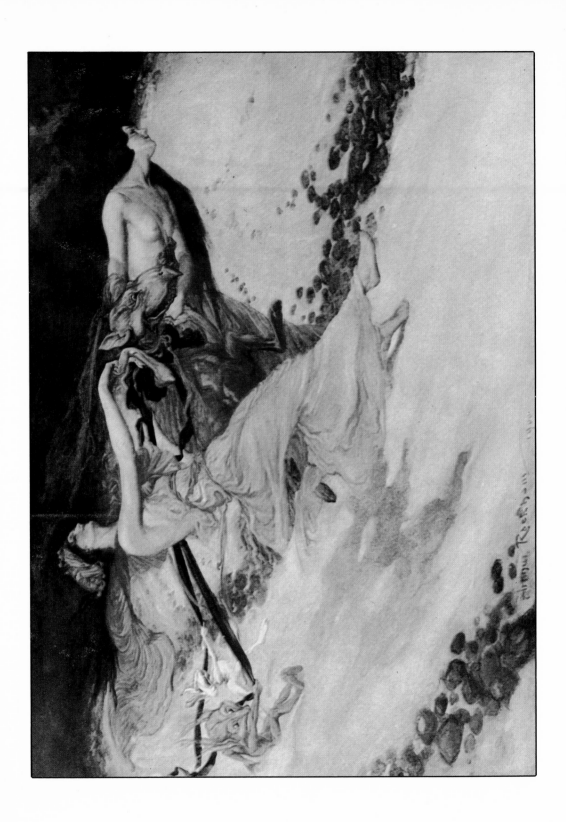

26   *Elfin Revellers*

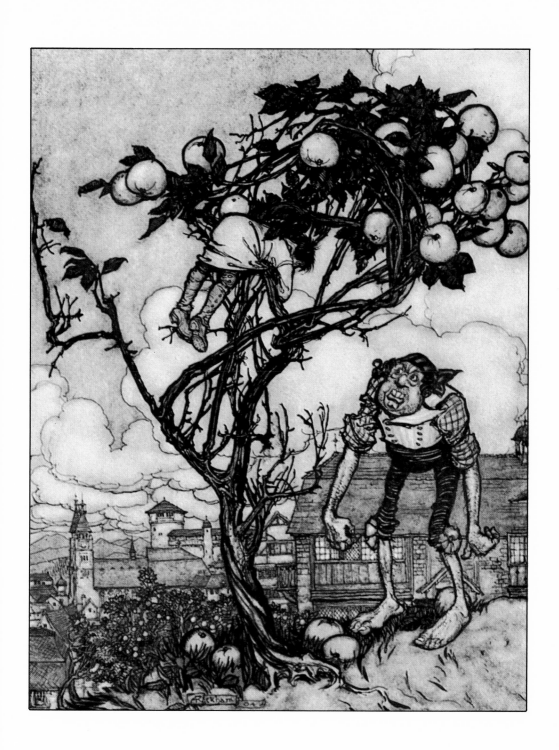

27   *Hi! You up there*

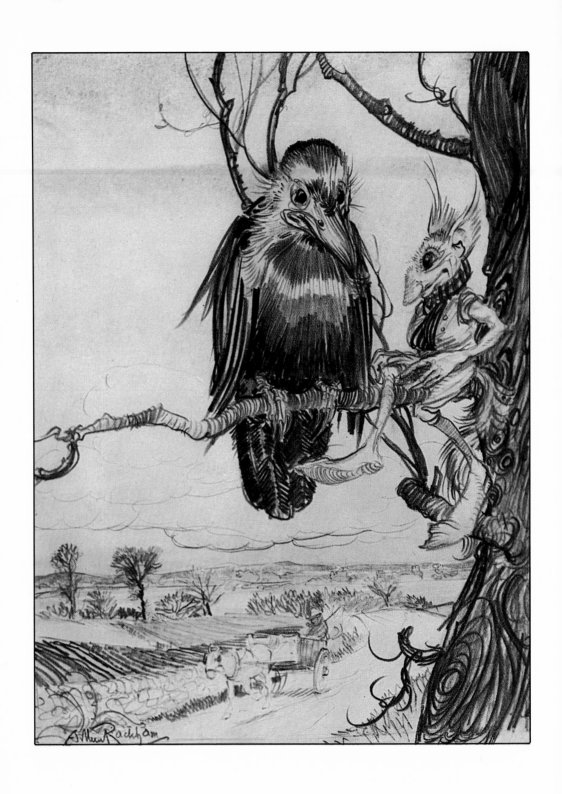

28   *The Gossips*

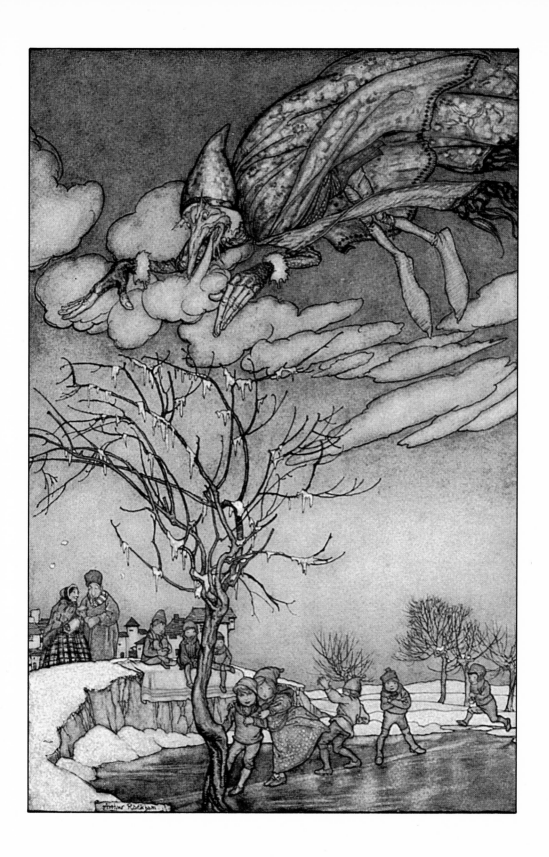

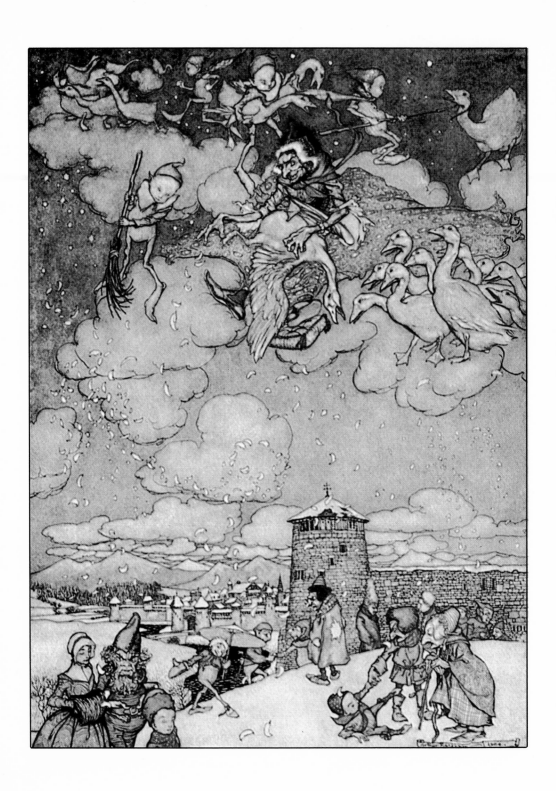

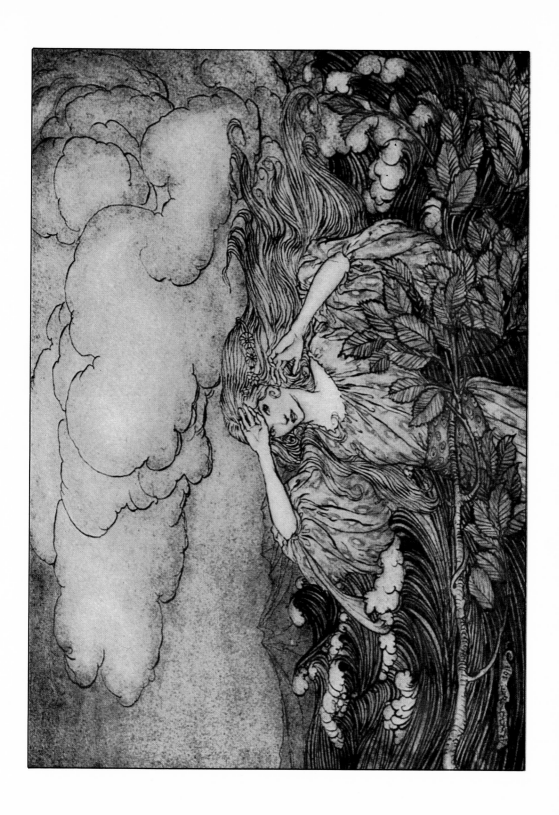

31   *The Wind and the Waves*

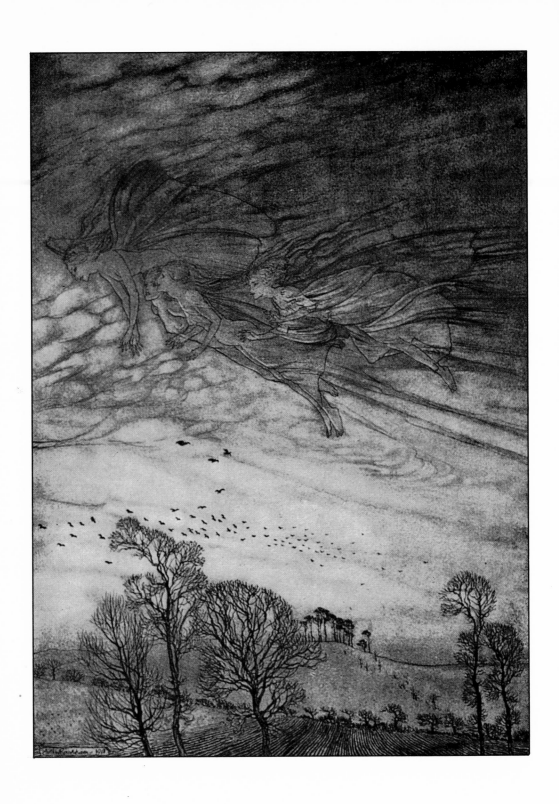

32   *Shades of Evening*

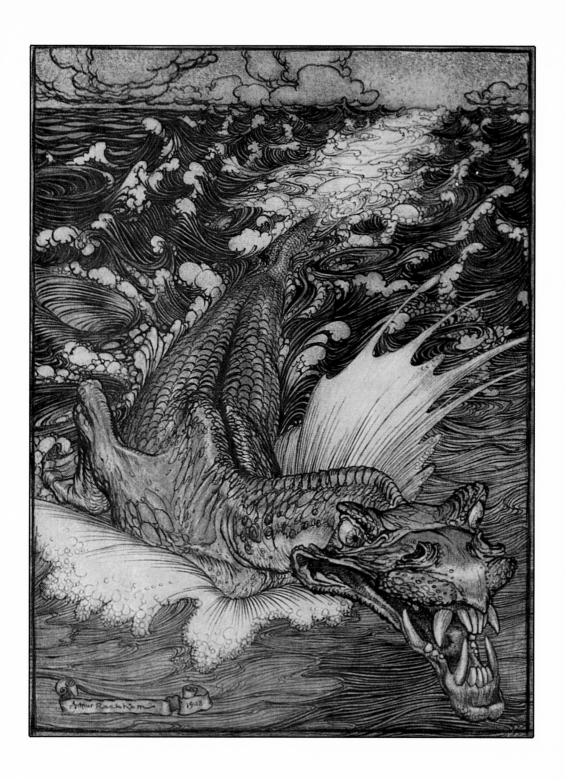

33   *The Leviathan*

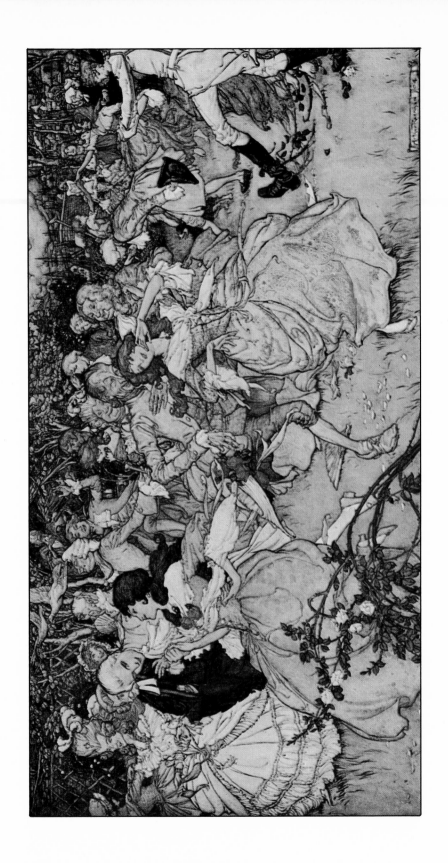

34   *Cupid's Alley*

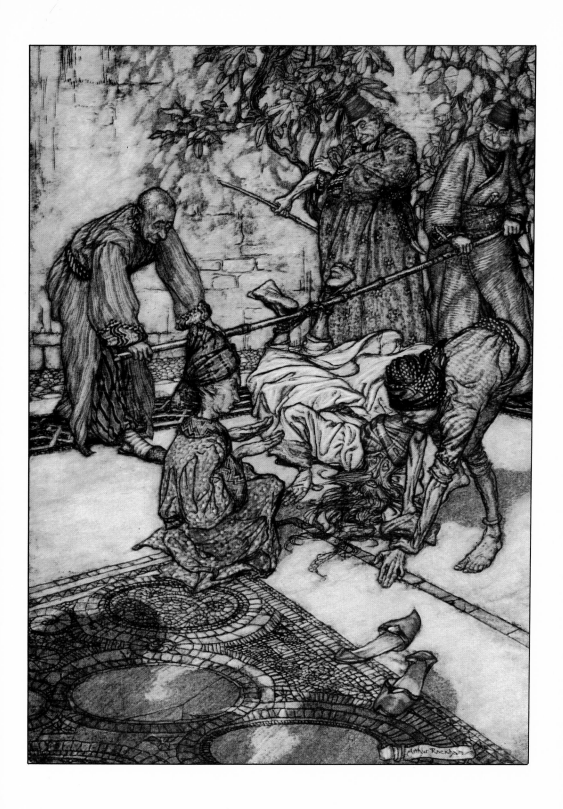

35   *Bastinado*

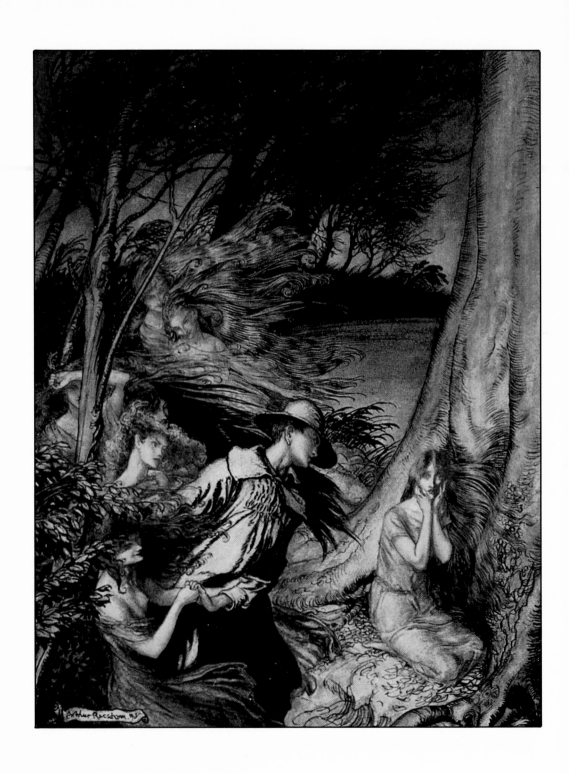